THE CANCER TECHNIQUES

SIMPLE PATTERNS FOR SURVIVING CANCER

DR. J. SIMON

Table of Contents

INTRODUCTION 3

CHAPTER ONE 6

   Risky Components...6

   The significance of cancer 9

   The Biology of Cancer 10

   Normal vs. Carcinogenic Cells 11

   Apoptosis, also known as programmed cell death: 14

   The formation of angiogenesis 14

   Common Risk Factors.................................15

   AGE...16

CHAPTER TWO 20

   Cancer Types 20

   Signs and Causes of Concern.....................23

   Verification...28

   Autopsies 29

   Laboratory examinations and pathology: 30

   Setting Up and Grading..............................32

   Options for Treatment 35

   Assistive Healthcare 40

CHAPTER THREE 43

Survival and Aftercare 45

Preventive Techniques 50

nutritious diet 51

Conclusion 56

THE END 59

INTRODUCTION

Unchecked development and spread of aberrant cells characterize cancer, a complex and multifaceted collection of disorders. These abnormal cells have the ability to invade nearby tissues and organs and destroy them. Cancer comes in a multitude of forms, each with distinct characteristics and tendencies that can impact nearly any area of the body.

Vital information regarding cancer includes:

Abnormalities within the cell

When genetic abnormalities cause uncontrollably rapid cell growth, normal cells can turn cancerous. These changes may be brought about by a variety of factors, including a genetic susceptibility, exposure to carcinogens, or other environmental effects.

Development of tumors

Masses or lumps known as tumors arise when aberrant cells continue to grow unchecked. Tumors can be malignant (cancerous) or benign (non-cancerous). Malignant tumors can spread to other parts of the body through the lymphatic or circulatory systems after invading nearby tissues.

Distribute:

Cancer cells have the ability to metastasize, or spread to new locations. The prognosis is usually worse and treatment for metastatic cancer is more challenging. Cancer cells can metastasize, resulting in tumors in distant organs.

Kinds of Cancer:

There are currently over a hundred different types of cancer, and they are all derived from specific tissues or organs. Prostate, colorectal, lung, breast, and leukemia cancers are among the prevalent types.

CHAPTER ONE

Risky Components

Cancer can develop due to a number of risk factors, including a person's genetic makeup, exposure to carcinogens (like tobacco smoke or UV radiation), unhealthy lifestyle choices (like eating poorly and not exercising), and certain infections.

Indices:

Depending on the type and stage of the disease, cancer symptoms can vary significantly. Frequently observed symptoms include lumps or tumors, persistent fatigue, irregular bleeding, altered bowel or bladder habits, and inexplicable weight loss.

The diagnostic process typically involves a combination of imaging studies, laboratory testing, and biopsy procedures. With the use of cutting-edge imaging techniques like CT, MRI, and PET scans, the location and extent of a tumor can be identified.

Situation:

Cancer is staged in order to determine the extent of its dissemination. A prognosis is provided by staging, which also helps to guide therapy decisions. Phases range from Stage 0 (localized and in situ) to Stage IV (advanced and metastatic).

Treatment:

Immunotherapy, targeted therapy, chemotherapy, radiation therapy, surgery, and hormone therapy are among the cancer treatment options. The choice of therapy depends on the kind, stage, and unique features of the cancer.

Resilience and Support:

Thanks to advancements in cancer research and therapy, the survivability rate has increased. Cancer survivors might struggle with their physical and mental well-being, requiring ongoing care and observation.

Avoidance:

Preventive methods include making lifestyle adjustments such as eating a balanced diet, exercising frequently, giving up tobacco and excessive alcohol use, and getting screened often for early detection.

Though much work remains in the field of global health, advancements in research, treatment, and prevention can help those affected by the disease live longer and in better health.

The significance of cancer

The word "cancer" generally refers to a group of diseases characterized by the unchecked growth and spread of abnormal cells. These cells can develop into tumors that impede the normal function of organs or tissues. Different body parts can be affected by cancer, which can appear in a multitude of forms and subtypes. Due to the complexity and multifaceted nature of the illness, customized treatment regimens are usually necessary.

The Biology of Cancer

Cancer biology is the study of the systems and mechanisms that underlie the development, metastasis, and behavior of cancer cells. It looks at interactions between the immune system, aberrant cell signaling, the tumor microenvironment, and genetic abnormalities as well as the cellular and molecular causes of cancer.

Comprehending the fundamental reasons behind cancer, the mechanisms by which normal cells transform into malignant ones, and the factors influencing the growth and spread of cancer are the aims of research on cancer biology. This knowledge is necessary to develop immunotherapies, targeted therapies, and other interventions for the management or prevention of cancer.

In short, the aim of cancer biology is to gain a deeper understanding of the disease's cellular and molecular components to enable the development of more accurate therapeutics and diagnostics.

Normal vs. Carcinogenic Cells

Normal and malignant cells differ in a few important ways.

Cell Growth and Division:

The controlled cycle of growth, division, and apoptosis (cell death) that normal cells go through helps to maintain tissue integrity and function.

Carcinogenic cells proliferate rapidly and frequently create tumors as a result of unchecked and aberrant cell proliferation.

Cellular Signaling:

Normal cell growth and division are regulated by bodily signals.

Cancer cells may become resistant to normal regulatory cues and instead promote uncontrolled growth as a result of modifications in their signaling pathways.

The composition of cells:

The structure of a typical cell is clear-cut and ordered.

Cancer cells often have abnormal nuclei, sizes, and shapes, which are signs of unchecked growth.

Deterrent Against Making Contact:

When normal cells come into contact with adjacent cells, a process known as contact inhibition causes the cells to stop dividing.

Cancer cells have the ability to aggregate into dense masses known as tumors because they may not show contact inhibition.

Apoptosis, also known as programmed cell death:

Apoptosis, a process that kills off healthy cells when they are no longer needed or destroyed, prevents the growth of abnormal cells.

Because they are resistant to death, cancer cells can live and multiply indefinitely.

The formation of angiogenesis

Only when necessary do normal cells stimulate angiogenesis, the growth of new blood vessels.

Cancer cells can initiate angiogenesis to sustain their own growth and survival as well as to supply blood.

It is crucial to understand these differences in order to develop customized treatments that target the unique characteristics of cancer cells with precision while minimizing harm to healthy cells.

Common Risk Factors

There are several common risk factors associated with an increased chance of developing cancer. Recall that some cancer patients may not have any clear-cut risk factors, and that having one or more risk factors does not guarantee that cancer will manifest. A few common risk factors are as follows:

The risk of cancer increases with age due to the cumulative effects of genetic changes.

Usage of Tobacco:

A considerable risk of lung, mouth, throat, and pancreatic cancers, among other cancers, is associated with smoking and using tobacco products.

Background in Family:

A family history of a particular cancer may increase one's risk, especially if close relatives were young when they were diagnosed with the disease.

Molecular Biology:

Inherited genetic changes, such as those connected to ovarian and breast cancer (BRCA genes), may raise an individual's risk of developing cancer.

Diet and Physical Activity:

It has been shown that obesity, a poor diet, and inactivity increase the risk of several cancers.

Solar Radiation Absorption:

Exposure to ultraviolet (UV) radiation from the sun or tanning beds increases the risk of skin cancer.

Aspects of the Environment:

Exposure to certain pollutants, toxins in the environment, and occupational hazards may raise one's risk of cancer.

Prolonged Inflammation:

Chronic inflammation, often associated with conditions such as inflammatory bowel disease, may increase a person's risk of developing certain cancers.

Consuming Alcohol:

An increased risk of liver, breast, and digestive system cancers has been associated with abnormal alcohol consumption.

Agents that Contain:

A number of bacteria and viruses, such as Helicobacter pylori, hepatitis B and C, and the human papillomavirus (HPV), can increase the risk of developing specific cancers.

It is imperative to bear in mind that various risk factors may interact with one another and that multiple factors may contribute to the development of cancer. A person's chance of getting some cancers can also be decreased by adopting preventative measures and altering their lifestyle. Regular testing and early detection are other essential components of cancer risk management.

CHAPTER TWO

Cancer Types

Cancer can take many different forms, and it can originate from any type of body tissue or cell. These are some of the common types of cancer:

Breast cancer: A disease that begins in the cells that comprise the breast tissue, it can strike both men and women.

Lung cancer: Typically brought on by tobacco use, lung cancer affects smokers but can also affect non-smokers.

Colorectal cancer: This condition typically affects the colon or the rectum and begins as polyps with the potential to spread to become malignant.

Prostate cancer is a disease that develops in the prostate gland of the male reproductive system.

Ovarian cancer is a disease that affects the ovaries in the female reproductive system.

A blood cancer that harms bone marrow and blood cells is called leukemia.

Pancreatic cancer starts to grow in the organ that produces insulin and digests enzymes, the pancreas.

Skin cancer: Contains both non-melanoma and melanoma types; UV radiation exposure is a common cause.

Forms in the lining of the bladder: Bladder cancer.

The kidneys, which are in charge of producing urine and filtering blood, are where kidney cancer begins to grow.

Chronic liver problems are often associated with liver cancer, a disease that originates in the liver cells.

Tumors that originate in the thyroid gland and impact the body's metabolism are referred to as thyroid cancers.

Brain cancer: It can originate in the brain, travel to other bodily parts, and impact various brain regions.

A type of lymphoma that impacts the lymphatic system is called Hodgkin's lymphoma.

Another lymphoma connected to the lymphatic system is non-Hodgkin's lymphoma.

These represent just a few of the many types of cancer; each has unique characteristics, causative agents, and therapeutic approaches. Advances in research are improving our understanding of cancer, leading to more accurate diagnosis methods and targeted treatments.

Signs and Causes of Concern

Numerous signs and symptoms may be connected to a given disease, depending on its type, location, and stage. However, there are a few typical signs and symptoms that may indicate cancer. It's important to keep in mind that these symptoms are not exclusive to cancer. It is advisable to consult a medical specialist for a thorough evaluation in case your symptoms worsen or stay the same. Typical symptoms and signs consist of the following:

Weight Loss Unexpectedly:

Sudden, unexplained weight loss that is significant could be a sign of one of several cancers.

Fatigued:

If you experience a chronic lack of strength and energy that does not improve with rest, it may be cancerous.

Affected:

Pain that doesn't go away with medicine or that is chronic and has no apparent cause could be cancer.

Alterations in the Skin:

Skin changes such as darkening, yellowing (jaundice), or changes in the appearance of moles may be reason for concern.

Changes to the Bowel or Bladder Habits:

Urinary tract or colorectal cancers may be indicated by persistent changes in bowel habits, such as diarrhea or constipation, and changes in bladder function.

Not Able to Swallow:

The inability to swallow, or dysphagia, is a symptom of esophageal or throat cancers.

Prolonged Cough or Rough Voice:

A persistent cough, hoarseness, or changes in voice could be signs of lung or throat cancer.

Bulges or swellings:

Unidentified lumps or swellings in the body that might be signs of cancer include breast lumps and testicular masses, for instance.

Menstrual pattern modifications:

Changes in menstrual patterns, such as heavy bleeding or irregular periods, may be associated with gynecological malignancies.

Breathing Problems:

Breathing difficulties or ongoing dyspnea may indicate lung cancer or other respiratory cancers.

A spike in temperature:

A specific type of cancer may be indicated by a persistent fever with unknown causes.

Sweats at night:

Anxiety-inducing, severe night sweats could indicate lymphoma or other cancers.

It is noteworthy to acknowledge that these symptoms may also be produced by non-cancerous illnesses. Regular health exams and screenings, as well as prompt medical attention when symptoms are concerning, help to improve outcomes and detect problems early.

Cancer is diagnosed using a variety of methods, including imaging scans, lab work, physical examinations, reviews of medical histories, and frequently a biopsy. Below is a summary of the diagnostic process:

Health History and Physical Examination:

The patient's symptoms, family history, and previous medical history will all be questioned by the medical expert. Another option would be to perform a thorough physical examination.

Imaging Study:

A range of imaging tests, such as CT, MRI, PET, and ultrasound, can be used to view internal structures and find any abnormalities or masses.

Blood Analysis:

Blood tests can be used to detect blood cell count abnormalities, pinpoint particular markers associated with particular cancers, or assess overall health.

Autopsies

A biopsy is a crucial initial procedure in the diagnosis of cancer. To be examined in a laboratory, a small sample of tissue from the alleged cancerous area needs to be extracted.

Many methods can be used to take biopsies, including endoscopic treatments, needle biopsies, and surgical biopsies.

A pathology facility receives the biopsy sample and examines it under a microscope. Pathologists inspect the tissue in order to determine the type of cancer, its grade, and other important details.

Analysis of Genes:

In certain situations, genetic testing may be recommended to identify specific genetic mutations or markers associated with an increased risk of developing a particular cancer. In certain cases, this can lead to targeted therapy, and in other cases, it can help direct treatment decisions.

Situation:

A crucial stage in staging is figuring out how far the cancer has spread. This information informs treatment decisions. Staging may require additional imaging studies and, in some cases, a surgical investigation.

Group Talk:

A multidisciplinary team of oncologists, radiologists, surgeons, and other experts can develop an appropriate treatment plan after reviewing the diagnostic data.

Accurately determining the type, stage, and other relevant details of the cancer is the aim of the diagnostic process. Following confirmation of the diagnosis, conversations regarding available treatments such as immunotherapy, radiation therapy, chemotherapy, surgery, or a combination of these can start. An correct diagnosis and early detection are essential for increasing the likelihood that cancer therapy will be successful.

Setting Up and Grading

Two crucial components of cancer characterization are staging and grading, which provide information about the severity and course of the disease and influence therapy choices.

Situation:

Finding the location and degree of cancer's spread inside the body is known as staging. The TNM system is the most widely used staging system.

Tumor (T): Indicates the primary tumor's dimensions.

Node (N): Shows if adjacent lymph nodes have been affected by malignancy.

Metastasis (M): Shows if cancer has extended to distant tissues or organs.

Roman numerals (I–IV) are commonly used to indicate staging; higher numbers denote more advanced disease. For instance, Stage IV tumors have spread to other bodily areas, whereas Stage I cancers are often tiny and contained.

Rating:

Grading is based on how cancer cells seem under the microscope and how differentiated they are (i.e., how similar they are to normal cells). The objective is to estimate the rate of growth and dissemination of the cancer cells.

For prostate cancer, the most widely used grading scheme is the Gleason score; for other malignancies, the World Health Organization (WHO) uses a different grading scheme. There are three common classifications for grading: badly differentiated (high grade), moderately differentiated (middle grade), and well differentiated (low grade).

High-grade tumors can contain abnormal-looking cells and have a tendency to grow more quickly than low-grade cancers, which typically have cells that resemble normal cells and are less aggressive.

For figuring out the prognosis and creating a suitable treatment strategy, staging and grading are both essential. By customizing treatments to the unique features of each malignancy, medical providers might increase the chances of favorable results by using the information gathered from these assessments.

Options for Treatment

Treatment for cancer is different depending on the patient's unique circumstances, the type of disease, and its stage. Typical forms of treatment consist of:

Surgery:

A typical strategy is surgical excision of the tumor or damaged tissue, particularly in cases with confined malignancies. It could be a part of a multimodal therapy approach or be curative.

Chemotherapy:

Drugs are used in chemotherapy to either kill or stop the growth of cancer cells. It can be used either alone or in conjunction with other treatments, and it can be given orally or intravenously.

Radiation Treatment:

High-energy beams are used in radiation therapy to target and kill cancer cells. It can be administered internally (brachytherapy) or externally (external beam radiation).

Immunotherapy:

The goal of immunotherapy is to strengthen the body's ability to identify and combat cancerous cells. Checkpoint inhibitors, CAR-T cell therapy, and other immune-strengthening medications are among them.

Hormone Treatment:

Cancers that are susceptible to hormones, like those of the breast and prostate, are treated with hormone therapy. It entails inhibiting or lessening the impact of hormones that promote specific forms of cancer.

Personalized Medicine:

Targeted therapies target particular molecules that are involved in the development and spread of cancer. These medications try to stop the signals that support the growth and division of cancer cells.

Stem Cell Transplantation:

Leukemia and lymphoma are two blood malignancies that may be candidates for stem cell transplantation. It entails grafting healthy stem cells into bone marrow that has been damaged or sick.

Precision Health Care:

Customizing a patient's course of treatment according to the unique genetic features of their cancer is known as precision medicine. Genetic testing to determine targeted treatments may be part of this.

Hospice Care:

Palliative care is centered on symptom relief, enhancing quality of life, and offering patients and their families support. It is compatible with restorative therapies.

Clinical Examinations:

By taking part in clinical trials, patients can benefit from cutting-edge treatments and further the field of cancer research.

Individualized treatment programs are common, and a mix of these methods may be employed. The objective is to attain the optimal result, which may entail treating the cancer with supportive care, stopping its spread, or curing it. A diverse healthcare team collaborates with the patient to make treatment decisions.

Assistive Healthcare

Palliative care, sometimes referred to as supportive care, aims to alleviate the symptoms and side effects of cancer and its treatment. It seeks to enhance the patient's and their family's quality of life. The following are essential elements of cancer supportive care:

Pain Control:

The main priority is treating and controlling discomfort associated with cancer. To reduce pain, therapies such as nerve blocks and medications may be employed.

Control of Symptoms:

It's critical to manage side effects of cancer and its treatments, including nausea, exhaustion, and dyspnea.

Psychological and Emotional Assistance:

Patients can manage the emotional effects of cancer with the use of psychological and emotional assistance. Counseling, therapy, and support groups might be part of this.

Support for Nutrition:

Sustaining a healthy diet is essential for general wellbeing. There may be nutritional help offered, such as dietary advice and supplementation.

Rehabilitation and Physical Therapy:

In addition to addressing mobility issues that may develop during and after cancer treatment, physical therapy can assist patients in maintaining or regaining their physical function.

Alternative Medicines:

Acupuncture, massage, and yoga are examples of complementary therapies that may be provided to help with symptom management and overall wellbeing.

CHAPTER THREE

Care During the End of Life:

End-of-life care for patients with advanced cancer centers on comfort, dignity, and support. To improve the last phases of life, hospice care may be taken into consideration.

Support for Decision-Making and Communication:

It is essential to support candid and open communication between patients, families, and healthcare professionals. Making decisions about end-of-life care and treatment alternatives with knowledge is supported.

Spiritual Assist:

A key component of supportive care can include attending to patients' spiritual needs and offering assistance to families within the framework of their religious convictions.

Coordination of Care:

Bringing together various healthcare experts to coordinate care guarantees a thorough and well-coordinated approach to addressing the patient's needs.

Supportive care providers, who may include palliative care doctors, nurses, social workers, and other medical specialists, frequently work in tandem with the primary oncology team to deliver care. It can be started at any point during the cancer journey and is not just restricted to end-of-life care. The intention is to improve the general quality of life for cancer patients as well as their capacity to manage the practical, psychological, and physical difficulties that come with their condition.

Survival and Aftercare

The physical, psychological, and practical problems that cancer survivors may experience following the conclusion of active treatment are the main focus of survivorship care. In order to manage any potential long-term effects of therapy, keep an eye on the patient's health, and handle any unresolved issues, follow-up care is a crucial part of survival. The following are important facets of cancer survivorship and aftercare:

Plans for Survivorship Care:

A survivorship care plan is a customized document that includes suggestions for follow-up care, possible long-term effects, and a description of the patient's cancer treatment. Information about healthy living choices might also be included.

Keep an Eye Out for Recurrence:

Frequent monitoring and follow-up consultations are essential to identify and treat any early indications of cancer recurrence. This could entail blood testing, imaging studies, and other evaluations depending on the particular cancer type and treatment history.

Handling Long-Term Repercussions:

Taking care of any long-term psychological or physical repercussions that cancer and its treatment may have is part of survivorship care. This might entail treating problems like exhaustion, altered cognition, and hormone abnormalities.

Psychosocial Assistance:

In order to address the psychological and emotional aspects of survivorship, it is critical to offer continuous psychosocial care. Support groups, counseling, and other services can assist survivors in overcoming obstacles they may encounter.

Promotion of a Healthful Lifestyle:

It is crucial to help and encourage survivors in establishing and upholding a healthy lifestyle. Advice on diet, exercise, quitting smoking, and other health-promoting practices is included in this.

Taking Care of Late Effects:

The body may experience late or delayed effects from some cancer treatments. Survivorship care is keeping an eye on and controlling these consequences, which could include heart problems, recurrent malignancies, or other problems.

Sexual Health and Fertility:

As part of survivorship care, conversations regarding sexual and reproductive health may take place. Family planning advice may also be given, along with potential effects of cancer therapy on reproductive health.

Coordination of Care:

In order to guarantee a thorough approach to survivorship, care coordination amongst different healthcare professionals is essential. Collaboration between primary care physicians, oncologists, and other specialists may be necessary for this.

Resources for Education:

Giving survivors access to educational materials and data keeps them informed about their health, possible hazards, and available resources for support.

The field of survivorship care is developing and is aware of the special requirements of cancer patients. The intention is to address any unresolved issues pertaining to their cancer journey while enabling survivors to lead healthy and meaningful lives after treatment. Personalized and successful survivorship care depends on regular communication between survivors and their medical team.

Preventive Techniques

Although there are some cancers that cannot be prevented, there are a number of ways to lower your risk of getting cancer. Here are a few crucial preventative techniques:

Changes in Lifestyle:

Give Up Smoking: One of the best strategies to lower your risk of developing any type of cancer, especially lung cancer, is to give up smoking.

Limit Alcohol Consumption: It is recommended to moderate alcohol intake as it has been associated with an increased risk of certain cancers.

nutritious diet

Eating a diet rich in fruits, vegetables, whole grains, lean meats, and other nutrients can improve general health and lower the risk of cancer.

Engaging in Exercise:

Regular physical activity has been linked to a decreased risk of various cancers. Try to get in at least 150 minutes a week of moderate-to-intense exercise.

Protection from the Sun:

Wearing protective clothes, applying sunscreen, and limiting your time outside in the sun can all help shield your skin from damaging UV radiation. This lowers the chance of developing skin cancer.

Immunization:

There are vaccines available to prevent some infections linked to a higher risk of cancer. The HPV vaccine, for instance, aids in preventing infections that may result in cervical and other cancers.

Early detection and screening:

Regular screenings can help identify cancer at earlier, more manageable stages. Examples of these screenings include mammograms, Pap smears, colonoscopies, and prostate cancer screenings.

Genetic Testing and Counseling:

Genetic testing and counseling may be beneficial for people with known genetic mutations or a family history of specific cancers. In assessing and managing the risk of hereditary cancers, this can be helpful.

Environmental and Occupational Safety:

Reduce your exposure to radon, asbestos, and other chemicals, as well as other environmental and occupational carcinogens. Observe safety precautions when working.

Prevention of Infections:

Prevent infections that have been connected to a higher risk of cancer by taking preventative measures. This entails using safe sexual practices, receiving hepatitis B and C vaccinations, and lowering one's risk of HIV.

Keep Your Weight in Check:

Numerous cancers are linked to an increased risk of being overweight or obese. A balanced diet and consistent exercise can aid in maintaining a healthy weight.

Hormone Replacement Therapy (HRT) Limitations:

In postmenopausal women, hormone replacement therapy has been linked to an increased risk of some cancers. Consult a healthcare professional about the possible risks and benefits of HRT if you're thinking about it.

It's crucial to remember that while these preventative techniques are generally advised, specific risks may differ. Screenings, regular check-ups with medical professionals, and leading a healthy lifestyle are all parts of a comprehensive cancer prevention plan.

Conclusion

In summary, cancer is a multifaceted group of illnesses defined by the unchecked division and proliferation of aberrant cells. It is a major global cause of morbidity and mortality and can affect any part of the body. Improvements in early detection, diagnosis, and treatment options have been made possible by advances in healthcare and research, even though not all cancers can be prevented.

Cancer risk can be decreased by taking preventive measures like leading a healthy lifestyle, abstaining from tobacco and excessive alcohol use, wearing sunscreen, and receiving vaccinations against certain infections. Frequent screenings, genetic testing, and family history knowledge are important factors in early detection, which enables more efficient treatment.

While there are many different approaches to treating cancer, surgery, chemotherapy, radiation therapy, immunotherapy, and targeted therapy are frequently used. Following active treatment, survivorship and follow-up care address the practical, emotional, and physical challenges that people with cancer face. They are crucial parts of the cancer journey.

Research that never stops, medical breakthroughs, and a multidisciplinary approach to cancer treatment keep improving results and raising the standard of living for cancer patients. To effectively manage and prevent cancer, people must remain informed, get regular checkups, and collaborate with healthcare professionals. It is hoped that with ongoing research, treatment, and prevention initiatives, the impact of cancer on people and communities around the world will be further diminished.

THE END

www.ingramcontent.com/pod-product-compliance
Lightning Source LLC
Chambersburg PA
CBHW060843260726
48661CB00002B/585